The Journey to Health

A Comprehensive Guide to Weight Loss

Alexandra Wells

Table of Contents

- Setting realistic expectations for progress

Chapter 3: Nutrition Essentials

- Exploring the basics of nutrition
- Understanding macronutrients (carbohydrates, proteins, fats) and micronutrients (vitamins, minerals)
- Knowledge about portion control and prudent eating
- Discussing the role of hydration in weight loss
- Tips for making healthier food choices

Chapter 4: Meal Planning and Preparation

- The importance of meal planning in weight loss
- Strategies for meal prepping to save time and stay on track
- Creating balanced and nutritious meals
- Incorporating variety and flavor into your diet
- Tips for dining out while still making healthy choices

Chapter 5: Exercise and Physical Activity

- Exploring the benefits of exercise for weight loss and overall health
- Designing a personalized exercise routine
- Incorporating cardiovascular, strength training, and flexibility exercises
- Tips for staying motivated and overcoming exercise barriers
- Discussing the importance of rest and recovery

Chapter 6: Mindset and Motivation

- Understanding the psychology of weight loss
- Techniques for staying inspired and overcoming setbacks
- Cultivating an optimistic body image and self-esteem
- Tips for managing stress and emotional eating
- Practicing mindfulness and self-compassion

- Celebrating milestones and non- scale victories.

- Staying flexible and adaptable

Chapter 10: Sustainable Habits for Long-Term Success

- Understanding sustainable habits

- Strategies for establishing sustainable habits

- The benefits of sustainable habits

Chapter 11: The Power of Self-reflection and Continuous Improvement

- Understanding self-reflection

- Benefits of self-reflection in weight loss

- Strategies for self-reflection

- Embracing continuous improvement

Appendix:

- Sample meal plans and recipes

- Exercise routines for beginners, intermediate, and advanced levels

- Glossary of terms commonly used in weight loss and nutrition

Introduction

This comprehensive guide provides readers with the knowledge, tools, and strategies they need to embark on a successful weight loss journey and achieve lasting results. By focusing on sustainable habits, mindset, and holistic wellness, individuals can overcome obstacles and transform their lives for the better.

Chapter 1: Understanding Weight Loss

In today's modern world, the pursuit of weight loss has become a prevalent goal for millions of individuals worldwide. It's a journey embarked upon by people from all walks of life, motivated by a desire to improve their health, enhance their physical appearance, or simply feel better in their own bodies. However, before delving into any weight loss endeavor, it's imperative to develop a deep understanding of what weight loss truly entails and the factors that contribute to its success.

Introduction to the Concept of Weight Loss

Weight loss, in its simplest definition, refers to the process of reducing one's body weight. This reduction typically involves the loss of body fat, although it can also encompass the loss of muscle mass and water weight. While weight loss is often associated with achieving a certain aesthetic ideal, its significance extends far beyond superficial appearances. At its core, weight loss is about optimizing one's overall health and well-being, reducing the risk of chronic diseases, and improving quality of life.

Exploring the Importance of Maintaining a Healthy Weight

Maintaining a healthy weight is paramount for ensuring optimal physical and mental health. Excess weight places undue strain on the body's organs and systems, increasing the risk of developing a myriad of health conditions, including diabetes, cardiovascular disease, hypertension, and certain types of cancer. Moreover, carrying excess weight can impair mobility, diminish energy levels, and negatively impact self-esteem and body image. By achieving and maintaining a healthy weight, individuals can enhance their vitality, longevity, and overall quality of life.

Debunking Common Myths About Weight Loss

In the realm of weight loss, misinformation and misconceptions abound, leading many individuals astray in their quest for a healthier body. From crash diets promising rapid results to the notion of "magic" weight loss supplements, separating fact from fiction is essential for success. One of the most pervasive myths is the belief that weight loss is solely a matter of willpower and calorie restriction. In reality, sustainable weight loss requires a multifaceted approach that encompasses nutrition, physical activity, stress management, sleep hygiene, and behavioral change. By dispelling common myths and embracing evidence-based strategies, individuals can navigate their weight loss journey with clarity and confidence.

Understanding the Science Behind Weight Gain and Loss

Weight gain and loss are governed by the fundamental principle of energy balance: when calorie intake exceeds calorie expenditure, the body stores excess energy as fat, leading to weight gain, whereas when calorie expenditure exceeds calorie intake, the body taps into its fat reserves for energy, resulting in weight loss. However, the process is far more complex than a simple equation of calories in versus calories out. Numerous factors influence weight regulation, including genetics, metabolism, hormonal fluctuations, gut health, environmental factors, and psychological variables such as stress, emotions, and habits. Understanding the intricate interplay of these factors is key to devising effective weight loss strategies tailored to individual needs and circumstances.

Discussing the Role of Metabolism in Weight Management

Metabolism, often misconstrued as a static entity, is a dynamic and multifaceted process that governs the body's energy expenditure and utilization. While some individuals may possess a naturally faster metabolism than others, metabolism is highly influenced by factors such as age, gender, body composition, genetics, dietary habits, physical activity levels, and hormonal balance. Contrary to popular belief, metabolism is not solely determined by genetics and cannot be drastically altered through quick-fix solutions or extreme measures. Rather, metabolism can be optimized and enhanced through lifestyle modifications such as regular exercise, balanced nutrition, adequate sleep, stress reduction, and muscle-building activities. By adopting a holistic approach to metabolism management, individuals can support their weight loss efforts and cultivate a healthier, more resilient body.

In summary, understanding weight loss is not merely about shedding pounds on the scale—it's about comprehending the intricate interplay of biological, psychological, and environmental factors that influence body weight and composition. By dispelling myths, embracing evidence-based knowledge, and adopting a holistic approach to health and wellness, individuals can embark on a transformative journey towards sustainable weight loss and lasting vitality.

Chapter 2: Setting Realistic Goals

In the pursuit of weight loss, setting realistic and achievable goals is paramount to long-term success. Goals provide direction, motivation, and a framework for progress, helping individuals stay focused and committed to their journey. However, not all goals are created equal, and the key to success lies in setting goals that are specific, measurable, achievable, relevant, and time-bound (SMART). In this chapter, we will delve into the importance of goal setting and provide practical strategies for creating a personalized weight loss plan.

The Importance of Setting Achievable Goals

Achievable goals serve as stepping stones on the path to success, guiding individuals through incremental progress and milestones. When goals are unrealistic or overly ambitious, they can set individuals up for disappointment and frustration, ultimately undermining their motivation and adherence to their plan. By setting achievable goals that align with one's capabilities, resources, and lifestyle, individuals can build confidence, momentum, and resilience, setting the stage for sustainable progress.

Strategies for Setting SMART Goals

SMART goals provide a framework for setting objectives that are clear, actionable, and attainable. Let's break down each component:

- Specific: Goals should be clear and well-defined, answering the questions of what, why, and how. Instead of vague statements like "lose weight," specify the desired outcome, such as "lose 10 pounds in three months."

- Measurable: Goals should be quantifiable, allowing improvement to be followed and assessed. This could involve tracking weight loss using a scale, measuring body fat percentage, or monitoring changes in clothing size.

- Achievable: Goals should be realistic and within reach, taking into account one's current circumstances, resources, and limitations. It's important to set goals that stretch but do not overwhelm, allowing for steady progress and sustainable lifestyle changes.

- Relevant: Goals should be aligned with one's values, priorities, and long-term objectives. They should address specific areas of improvement related to weight loss, such as dietary habits, physical activity levels, or stress management techniques.

- Time-bound: Goals should have a defined timeline or deadline, creating a sense of urgency and accountability. Setting deadlines helps prevent procrastination and fosters a sense of focus and commitment to action.

Creating a Personalized Weight Loss Plan

Once SMART goals have been established, it's time to develop a personalized weight loss plan tailored to individual needs and preferences. This plan should incorporate evidence-based strategies for nutrition, exercise, behavior change, and self-care, with the flexibility to adapt as circumstances evolve. Elements of a comprehensive weight loss plan may include:

- Nutrition: Adopting a balanced and nutritious eating plan that emphasizes whole foods, lean proteins, fruits, vegetables, and whole grains while limiting processed foods, added sugars, and unhealthy fats.

- Exercise: Incorporating regular physical activity into daily life, including cardiovascular exercise, strength training, flexibility exercises, and activities that promote overall well-being and enjoyment.

- Behavior Change: Cultivating healthy habits, mindset shifts, and coping strategies to overcome obstacles, manage cravings, and navigate social and emotional triggers.

- Self-Care: Prioritizing rest, relaxation, and stress management techniques such as mindfulness, meditation, yoga, or deep breathing exercises to promote physical and mental well-being.

Setting Realistic Expectations for Progress

While setting goals is essential for motivation and direction, it's equally important to maintain realistic expectations for progress. Weight loss is not linear, and there will inevitably be ups and downs along the way. Plateaus, setbacks, and fluctuations are normal parts of the journey, and it's essential to approach them with patience, resilience, and self-compassion. By focusing on consistent effort, small victories, and long-term sustainability, individuals can achieve lasting success in their weight loss endeavors.

In summary, setting realistic and achievable goals is a crucial step in the weight loss journey, providing a roadmap for success and empowering individuals to take charge of their health and well-being. By embracing the principles of SMART goal setting, creating a personalized weight loss plan, and maintaining realistic expectations, individuals can embark on a transformative journey towards a healthier, happier, and more vibrant life.

Chapter 3: Nutrition Essentials

Nutrition lies at the heart of any successful weight loss journey. By understanding the fundamentals of nutrition and making informed food choices, individuals can fuel their bodies effectively, support their weight loss goals, and promote overall health and well-being. In this chapter, we'll explore the essential components of nutrition, delve into the importance of balanced eating, and provide practical tips for making healthier food choices.

Exploring the Basics of Nutrition

Nutrition is the science of how the body obtains and utilizes nutrients from food to support growth, repair, and metabolic functions. It encompasses macronutrients, which provide energy in the form of calories, and micronutrients, which are essential for various physiological processes. The three primary macronutrients are:

- Carbohydrates: The body's main source of energy, found in foods like grains, fruits, vegetables, and legumes.
- Proteins: Essential for building and repairing tissues, supporting immune function, and maintaining muscle mass. Sources include meat, poultry, fish, dairy, legumes, nuts, and seeds.
- Fats: Important for hormone production, cell membrane integrity, and absorption of fat-soluble vitamins. Nutritious sources of fat include avocados, nuts, seeds, olive oil, and fatty fish.

Micronutrients, including vitamins and minerals, play crucial roles in metabolism, immune function, bone health, and overall vitality. Consuming a diverse array of nutrient-dense foods is essential for meeting micronutrient needs and supporting optimal health.

Understanding Portion Control and Mindful Eating

Portion control is a key aspect of weight management, as consuming excessive portions can lead to overeating and weight gain. Practicing portion control involves being mindful of serving sizes and paying attention to hunger and fullness cues. Techniques such as measuring food portions, using smaller plates, and eating slowly can help individuals regulate their intake and prevent overconsumption.

Mindful eating is another valuable practice that encourages individuals to cultivate awareness and presence during meals. By paying attention to sensory experiences, such as taste, texture, and aroma, and tuning into hunger and satiety cues, individuals can develop a healthier relationship with food, prevent mindless eating, and savor the eating experience.

Learning About Portion Control and Mindful Eating

Meal planning and preparation are essential components of a successful weight loss plan, enabling individuals to make healthier food choices, control portions, and manage their calorie intake. When planning meals, it's helpful to incorporate a balance of macronutrients and include a variety of colorful fruits, vegetables, lean proteins, and whole grains. Batch cooking and meal prepping can save time and effort during busy weeks, making it easier to stick to healthy eating habits.

Discussing the Role of Hydration in Weight Loss

Hydration plays a crucial role in weight loss for several reasons:

- Appetite Control: Drinking water before meals can help reduce appetite, leading to fewer calorie intake during meals.

-Calorie-Free: Unlike sugary beverages, water is calorie-free, making it an excellent choice for staying hydrated without adding extra calories to your diet.

-Metabolism: Staying hydrated helps maintain proper metabolic function, which is essential for burning calories efficiently.

-Workout Performance: Being properly hydrated improves workout performance, allowing you to exercise more effectively and burn more calories.

-Water Retention: Adequate hydration can help prevent water retention, which can make you feel bloated and temporarily increase your weight.

Overall, staying hydrated is essential for overall health and can support weight loss efforts when combined with a balanced diet and regular exercise.

Tips for Making Healthier Food Choices

When navigating food choices, it's essential to prioritize nutrient-dense foods that provide essential nutrients without excess calories, sugar, or unhealthy fats. Some tips for making healthier food choices include:

- Opting for whole, minimally processed foods over highly processed and refined products.

- Reading food labels and ingredient lists to identify hidden sugars, unhealthy fats, and artificial additives.

- Choosing lean protein sources, such as poultry, fish, tofu, and legumes, instead of fatty cuts of meat.

- Incorporating plenty of fruits and vegetables into meals and snacks to boost fiber intake and promote satiety.

- Limiting intake of sugary beverages, including soda, fruit juices, and energy drinks, in favor of water, herbal tea, or infused water.

By adopting a balanced and mindful approach to nutrition, individuals can fuel their bodies effectively, support their weight loss goals, and lay the foundation for long-term health and vitality.

In summary, nutrition is a cornerstone of successful weight loss, providing the essential building blocks for energy, metabolism, and overall well-being. By understanding the basics of nutrition, practicing portion control and mindful eating, meal planning and preparation, hydration in weight loss, and making healthier food choices, individuals can nourish their bodies, achieve their weight loss goals, and thrive in their health journey.

Chapter 4: Meal Planning and Preparation

Meal planning and preparation are essential components of a successful weight loss journey. By taking the time to plan and prepare meals in advance, individuals can make healthier food choices, control portion sizes, and stay on track with their dietary goals. In this chapter, we'll explore the importance of meal planning and preparation, provide practical tips for getting started, and offer strategies for incorporating balanced and nutritious meals into daily life.

The Importance of Meal Planning

Meal planning involves deciding in advance what to eat for each meal and snack throughout the week. This proactive approach to eating not only saves time and reduces stress but also promotes healthier food choices and portion control. With a well-thought-out meal plan, individuals can ensure they have nutritious options on hand, minimize impulse eating, and avoid resorting to unhealthy convenience foods.

Strategies for Meal Prepping

Meal prepping goes hand in hand with meal planning and involves preparing meals or ingredients in advance to streamline the cooking process throughout the week. Some effective meal prepping strategies include:

- Batch cooking: Preparing large quantities of food at once, such as soups, stews, or casseroles, and portioning them into individual servings for easy reheating.
- Pre-cutting fruits and vegetables: Washing, chopping, and portioning fresh produce ahead of

time for quick and convenient snacks or meal additions.

- Preparing grab-and-go options: Making homemade snacks, such as energy balls, trail mix, or pre-portioned yogurt parfaits, for quick and healthy snacks on the go.

- Planning diverse ingredients: Choosing ingredients that can be used in numerous recipes throughout the week to minimize waste and maximize efficiency.

Creating Balanced and Nutritious Meals

When planning meals, it's important to prioritize balanced nutrition by including a variety of food groups and nutrients. A well-balanced meal typically consists of:

- Lean protein: Such as chicken, turkey, fish, tofu, beans, or lentils, which provide essential amino acids for muscle repair and satiety.

- Whole grains: Such as brown rice, quinoa, barley, or whole wheat pasta, which provide fiber, vitamins, and minerals for sustained energy.

- Vegetables: Such as leafy greens, broccoli, bell peppers, carrots, or tomatoes, which provide essential vitamins, minerals, and antioxidants.

- Healthy fats: Such as avocado, nuts, seeds, or olive oil, which provide essential fatty acids for heart health and nutrient absorption.

- Flavorful seasonings: Such as herbs, spices, citrus zest, or vinegar, to enhance the taste of meals without adding excess calories or sodium.

Incorporating Variety and Flavor

Variety is the spice of life, and it's essential for maintaining interest and enjoyment in healthy eating. Experimenting with different cuisines, flavors, and cooking techniques can make mealtime more exciting and satisfying. Some tips for incorporating variety and flavor into meals include:

- Trying new recipes: Exploring cookbooks, websites, or cooking apps for inspiration and trying out new recipes to keep meals interesting.
- Using herbs and spices: Experimenting with a variety of herbs, spices, and seasonings to add depth and flavor to dishes without excessive salt or fat.
- Incorporating global flavors: Exploring cuisines from around the world and incorporating ingredients and flavors from different cultures into meals.

Tips for Dining Out

While meal planning and preparation are valuable tools for controlling food choices and portions, there will inevitably be occasions when dining out is necessary or desired. In these situations, it's important to make mindful choices and prioritize nutritious options. Some tips for dining out while still making healthy choices include:

- Researching menus in advance: Reviewing restaurant menus online before dining out to identify healthier options and plan your meal in advance.
- Making substitutions: Requesting modifications to dishes, such as substituting steamed vegetables for French fries or asking for dressings and sauces on the side.
- Practicing portion control: Being mindful of portion sizes and avoiding oversized portions by sharing entrees or saving half for later.

In summary, meal planning and preparation are invaluable tools for supporting weight loss goals and promoting overall health and well-being. By taking a proactive approach to meal planning, incorporating balanced and nutritious ingredients, and embracing variety and flavor, individuals can enjoy delicious and satisfying meals while staying on track with their dietary objectives. Additionally, by practicing mindful choices when dining out, individuals can navigate social situations while still making progress towards their weight loss goals. With careful planning and preparation, eating healthily can be both convenient and enjoyable, making it easier to maintain a healthy lifestyle for the long term.

Chapter 5: Exercise and Physical Activity

Exercise is a vital segment of any successful weight loss journey. Not only does it help burn calories and promote fat loss, but it also improves overall health, boosts mood, and enhances quality of life. In this chapter, we'll explore the benefits of exercise, discuss different types of physical activity, and provide practical tips for incorporating exercise into daily life.

The Benefits of Exercise

Regular physical activity offers a wide range of benefits beyond weight loss. These include:

- Calorie expenditure: Exercise burns calories, helping create a calorie deficit necessary for weight loss.

- Improved metabolism: Regular exercise can boost metabolism, making it easier to maintain weight loss over time.

- Muscle preservation: Strength training helps preserve lean muscle mass, which is important for maintaining a healthy metabolism.

- Cardiovascular health: Aerobic exercise strengthens the heart and improves circulation, reducing the risk of heart disease.

- Mood enhancement: Exercise releases endorphins, chemicals that promote feelings of happiness and well-being, reducing stress and anxiety.

- Better sleep: Regular physical activity can improve sleep quality and duration, leading to better overall health and well-being.

Types of Physical Activity

There are several types of physical activity, each offering unique benefits:

- Cardiovascular exercise: Also known as aerobic exercise, this type of activity gets the heart rate up and increases breathing rate. Examples include walking, running, cycling, swimming, and dancing.

- Strength training: Strength training involves using resistance, such as weights or resistance bands, to build muscle mass and strength. It can include exercises such as weightlifting, bodyweight exercises, and resistance band workouts.

- Flexibility and mobility exercises: These exercises focus on improving flexibility, range of motion, and joint mobility. Examples include yoga, Pilates, and stretching routines.

- Functional training: Functional exercises mimic movements used in daily activities, such as squatting, bending, and lifting. They help improve balance, coordination, and stability.

Designing a Personalized Exercise Routine

When designing an exercise routine, it's important to consider individual fitness levels, goals, preferences, and any potential limitations or health concerns. A well-rounded exercise routine typically includes a combination of cardiovascular exercise, strength training, flexibility exercises, and functional movements.

Incorporating Exercise Into Daily Life

Incorporating exercise into daily life doesn't have to be complicated or time-consuming. There are numerous easy ways to increase physical training throughout the day, such as:

- Climbing the stairs rather than the elevators.
- Parking a little bit far from your destination and walking.

- Going for a walk during lunch breaks or after dinner.

- Doing bodyweight exercises while watching TV or listening to music.

- Taking up active hobbies such as gardening, dancing, or playing sports.

Staying Motivated and Overcoming Barriers

Staying motivated to exercise can be challenging, especially when faced with busy schedules, fatigue, or lack of motivation. Some strategies for staying motivated and overcoming barriers include:

- Setting realistic and achievable goals.
- Finding activities you enjoy and mixing up your routine to keep things interesting.
- Scheduling exercise sessions like appointments and treating them as non-negotiable.

- Enlisting the support of friends, family members, or workout buddies for accountability and encouragement.

- Being kind to yourself and acknowledging that progress takes time and effort.

The Importance of Rest and Recovery

Rest and recovery are essential components of any exercise program. Giving your body time to rest and repair itself between workouts helps prevent injury, reduce fatigue, and maximize performance. It's important to listen to your body's signals and prioritize adequate sleep, hydration, nutrition, and stress management for optimal recovery.

In summary, exercise is a critical aspect of weight loss and overall health, offering a myriad of benefits for physical, mental, and emotional well-being. By incorporating a variety of physical activities into daily life, designing a personalized exercise routine, staying motivated, and prioritizing rest and recovery, individuals can achieve their weight loss goals and enjoy the many rewards of an active lifestyle. With consistency, dedication, and a positive mindset, exercise can become a rewarding and sustainable part of daily life, leading to improved health and vitality for years to come.

Chapter 6: Mindset and Motivation

The journey to weight loss is not just about physical changes—it also involves a significant psychological component. Cultivating the right mindset and staying motivated are essential for overcoming challenges, staying on track, and achieving long-term success. In this chapter, we'll explore the psychology of weight loss, strategies for staying motivated, and techniques for maintaining a positive mindset throughout the journey.

Understanding the Psychology of Weight Loss

Weight loss is as much a mental and emotional journey as it is a physical one. Many factors influence our relationship with food, exercise, and our bodies, including past experiences, beliefs, emotions, and social influences. Understanding these psychological factors is key to addressing underlying issues, overcoming obstacles, and creating lasting change.

Strategies for Staying Motivated

Staying motivated can be challenging, especially when faced with setbacks or obstacles. Some strategies for staying motivated include:

- Setting meaningful goals: Identify goals that are personally meaningful and aligned with your values and priorities.
- Visualizing success: Visualize yourself achieving your goals and imagine how it will feel to reach them.
- Tracking progress: Keep track of your progress using tools such as a journal, progress photos, or fitness apps to celebrate victories and stay accountable.

- Rewarding yourself: Celebrate milestones along the way with non-food rewards, such as a new workout outfit, a massage, or a day off to relax.

- Finding support: Surround yourself with supportive friends, family members, or a community of like-minded individuals who can offer encouragement, advice, and accountability.

- Staying positive: Focus on the progress you've made rather than dwelling on setbacks, and practice self-compassion and kindness towards yourself.

Cultivating a Positive Body Image and Self-Esteem

Body image and self-esteem play a significant role in our motivation and behavior around food and exercise. Cultivating a positive body image involves accepting and appreciating your body for its strengths and capabilities, rather than focusing solely on its appearance. Some strategies for cultivating a positive body image include:

- Practicing self-care: Prioritize activities that make you feel good, whether it's taking a relaxing bath, spending time in nature, or indulging in a hobby you love.
- Surrounding yourself with positivity: Surround yourself with people, media, and environments that promote body positivity and self-acceptance.
- Challenging negative thoughts: Challenge negative thoughts and beliefs about your body by focusing on its functionality and what it allows you to do, rather than its appearance.
- Engaging in positive self-talk: Replace negative self-talk with positive affirmations and messages of self-love and acceptance.

Strategies for Managing Stress and Emotional Eating

Stress and emotions can trigger overeating or unhealthy eating habits, undermining weight loss efforts. Some strategies for managing stress and emotional eating include:

- Identifying triggers: Recognize the situations, emotions, or thoughts that trigger emotional eating and develop alternative coping strategies.
- Practicing mindfulness: Use mindfulness techniques, such as deep breathing, meditation, or yoga, to become more aware of your emotions and responses to stress.
- Finding healthy outlets: Find alternative ways to cope with stress or negative emotions, such as going for a walk, talking to a friend, or engaging in a creative activity.
- Searching for experienced help: If pressure or emotional eating becomes overwhelming, consider

searching for support from a therapist or consultant who can help you develop healthier coping means.

Practicing Mindfulness and Self-Compassion

Mindfulness and self-compassion are powerful tools for promoting emotional well-being and resilience on the weight loss journey. Some ways to incorporate mindfulness and self-compassion into your life include:

- Practicing gratitude: Take time each day to reflect on things you're grateful for and appreciate the positive aspects of your life.
- Being present: Practice being fully present in the moment, whether it's during meals, workouts, or daily activities, without judgment or distraction.
- Showing yourself kindness: Treat yourself with the same kindness and compassion you would show to a

friend, especially during times of difficulty or struggle.

- Accepting imperfection: Embrace the idea that perfection is unattainable and that setbacks and challenges are a natural part of the journey.

In summary, cultivating the right mindset and staying motivated are essential for success on the weight loss journey. By understanding the psychology of weight loss, setting meaningful goals, cultivating a positive body image and self-esteem, managing stress and emotional eating, and practicing mindfulness and self-compassion, individuals can overcome obstacles, stay focused, and achieve their goals with confidence and resilience. With a positive mindset and unwavering determination, anything is possible on the journey to a healthier, happier life.

Chapter 7: Sleep and Stress Management for Weight Loss

Sleep and stress management play crucial roles in weight loss and overall health. In this chapter, we'll explore the impact of sleep and stress on weight management, strategies for improving sleep quality and managing stress, and their importance in achieving long-term success.

The Importance of Sleep for Weight Loss

Quality sleep is essential for various aspects of health, including metabolism, hormone regulation, appetite control, and energy levels. Lack of sleep can disrupt these processes, leading to imbalances that contribute to weight gain and difficulty losing weight. Here's how poor sleep affects weight loss:

- Hormonal Imbalance: Sleep deprivation disrupts hormones that regulate hunger and appetite, such as ghrelin and leptin, leading to increased appetite and cravings for high-calorie foods.

- Metabolic Dysfunction: Sleep loss can impair glucose metabolism and insulin sensitivity, increasing the risk of insulin resistance and weight gain.

- Energy Levels: Inadequate sleep can leave you feeling tired and sluggish, making it harder to stay active and motivated to exercise.

- Emotional Eating: Lack of sleep can increase stress levels and emotional flux, leading to a tremendous tendency to turn to food for solace or stress relief.

Strategies for Improving Sleep Quality

Improving sleep quality is essential for supporting weight loss efforts and overall well-being. Here are some strategies to promote better sleep:

- Establish a Routine: Go to bed and wake up at the same time each day, even on weekends, to regulate your body's internal clock.

- Create a Relaxing Environment: Make your bedroom conducive to sleep by keeping it cool, dark, and quiet. Invest in a comfortable mattress and pillows.

- Limit Screen Time: Avoid electronic devices such as smartphones, tablets, and computers before bedtime, as the blue light can disrupt sleep patterns.

- Practice Relaxation Techniques: Wind down before bed with relaxation techniques such as deep breathing, meditation, or gentle stretching.

- Limit Stimulants: Avoid caffeine and nicotine in the hours leading up to bedtime, as they can interfere with sleep quality.

- Watch Your Diet: Avoid heavy meals, spicy foods, and excessive liquids close to bedtime, as they can cause discomfort and disrupt sleep.

The Impact of Stress on Weight Loss

Chronic stress can have a significant impact on weight management by influencing behaviors such as overeating, emotional eating, and sedentary lifestyle choices. Stress triggers the release of cortisol, a hormone that can increase appetite and promote fat storage, particularly around the abdomen. Additionally, stress can lead to poor sleep quality, further exacerbating weight-related issues.

Stress Management Strategies

Managing stress effectively is crucial for supporting weight loss and overall health. Here are some strategies for reducing stress:

- Exercise Regularly: Physical activity is a substantial stress reliever that releases endorphins and promotes ease. Strive for 30 minutes of standard exercise most days of the week.

- Practice Mindfulness: Mindfulness techniques such as meditation, deep breathing, and progressive muscle relaxation can help calm the mind and reduce stress levels.

- Set Boundaries: Learn to say no to excessive commitments and prioritize activities that bring you joy and relaxation.

- Seek Social Support: Lean on friends, family members, or support groups for emotional support and encouragement during stressful times.

- Maintain a Healthy Lifestyle: Eat a balanced diet, get regular exercise, and prioritize sleep to support your body's ability to cope with stress.

- Seek Professional Help: If stress becomes overwhelming or unmanageable, consider seeking support from a therapist or counselor who can provide strategies for coping with stress more effectively.

In summary, sleep and stress management are essential components of a successful weight loss journey. By prioritizing quality sleep, implementing strategies to improve sleep hygiene, and adopting stress management techniques, individuals can support their weight loss efforts and promote overall health and well-being. Remember that achieving sustainable weight loss requires a holistic approach that addresses not only diet and exercise but also sleep quality and stress levels. By taking care of your body and mind, you can set yourself up for long-term success and enjoy the many benefits of a healthier lifestyle.

Chapter 8: Overcoming Plateaus and Setbacks

Plateaus and setbacks are inevitable on the weight loss journey, but they don't have to derail your progress. In this chapter, we'll explore common reasons for plateaus and setbacks, provide strategies for overcoming them, and offer tips for staying resilient in the face of challenges.

Understanding Plateaus

Plateaus are periods of stalled progress or slower-than-expected weight loss despite continued efforts. They can be frustrating and demotivating, but they're a normal part of the weight loss process. Plateaus often occur when the body adapts to changes in diet and exercise, resulting in a temporary halt in weight loss. Other factors, such as hormonal fluctuations, stress, lack of sleep, and metabolic adaptation, can also contribute to plateaus.

Strategies for Overcoming Plateaus

When faced with a plateau, it's important to stay patient and persistent. Some strategies for overcoming plateaus include:

- Reassessing your habits: Take a closer look at your diet, exercise routine, and lifestyle habits to identify areas for improvement. Are you being consistent with your calorie intake and expenditure? Are you getting enough sleep and managing stress effectively?
- Mixing up your routine: Shake things up by trying new exercises, changing your workout intensity or duration, or experimenting with different types of physical activity. Variety can help prevent boredom and stimulate new progress.

- Adjusting your calorie intake: If you've been following the same calorie intake for a while, consider adjusting it slightly to create a calorie deficit. This could involve reducing portion sizes, increasing protein intake, or incorporating more low-calorie, nutrient-dense foods into your diet.

- Focusing on non-scale victories: Shift your focus away from the scale and celebrate other signs of progress, such as improvements in strength, endurance, energy levels, or body composition. These non-scale victories are just as important as the number on the scale.

- Seeking support: Reach out to a friend, family member, or support group for encouragement and accountability. Sharing your challenges and triumphs with others can provide valuable perspective and motivation.

Dealing with Setbacks

Setbacks are an inevitable part of any weight loss journey, but they don't have to define your success. Whether it's a minor slip-up or a major obstacle, setbacks provide an opportunity for growth and learning. Some strategies for dealing with setbacks include:

- Accepting imperfection: Accept that setbacks are a natural part of the process and that nobody is perfect. Instead of dwelling on mistakes, focus on what you can learn from them and how you can move forward.
- Practicing self-compassion: Be kind to yourself during challenging times and avoid self-criticism. Treat yourself with the same kindness and understanding you would show to a friend facing a similar situation.
- Recommitting to your goals: Use setbacks as motivation to recommit to your goals and redouble your efforts. Reflect on your reasons for wanting to

lose weight and reconnect with your inner sense of purpose and determination.

- Seeking support: Lean on your support network for encouragement, guidance, and accountability during times of struggle. Don't be afraid to ask for help when you need it, whether it's from friends, family, or a professional.

Staying Resilient

Resilience is the ability to rebound from lapses and challenges vigorous than before. Cultivating resilience is essential for long-term success on the weight loss journey. Some ways to build resilience include:

- Cultivating a growth mindset: Embrace challenges as opportunities for growth and learning rather than insurmountable obstacles. Adopting a growth mindset can help you approach setbacks with optimism and perseverance.

- Fostering gratitude: Focus on the positive aspects of your life and cultivate gratitude for the progress you've made, no matter how small. Gratitude can help shift your perspective and keep setbacks in perspective.

- Staying flexible: Remain open to new ideas, approaches, and strategies for overcoming challenges. Flexibility and adaptability are key qualities of resilient individuals.

- Practicing self-care: Prioritize self-care activities that nurture your physical, mental, and emotional well-being, such as exercise, relaxation techniques, hobbies, and social connections.

In summary, plateaus and setbacks are inevitable on the weight loss journey, but they don't have to derail your progress. By understanding the reasons behind plateaus, implementing strategies for overcoming them, and cultivating resilience in the face of setbacks, you can navigate the ups and downs of the journey with confidence and determination. Remember that setbacks are temporary, and with persistence, patience, and a positive mindset, you can overcome any obstacle and achieve your weight loss goals.

Chapter 9: Long-Term Maintenance and Sustainability

Achieving weight loss is a significant accomplishment, but maintaining those results in the long term is the ultimate goal. In this chapter, we'll explore strategies for transitioning from weight loss to weight maintenance, establishing sustainable habits, and embracing a healthy lifestyle for the long haul.

Transitioning to Maintenance Mode

Transitioning from weight loss to weight maintenance requires a shift in mindset and approach. While the focus during weight loss may have been on creating a calorie deficit and shedding pounds, maintenance involves finding a balance that allows you to sustain your results without feeling deprived or overwhelmed.

Setting Realistic Expectations

Maintaining weight loss is not about perfection but rather consistency and moderation. It's normal for weight to fluctuate slightly over time, and occasional indulgences or setbacks are part of a balanced lifestyle. Setting realistic expectations and accepting that progress may be slower or less linear than during the weight loss phase can help prevent frustration and disappointment.

Embracing Sustainable Habits

Sustainability is key to long-term success in weight maintenance. Instead of relying on short-term fixes or restrictive diets, focus on adopting sustainable habits that you can maintain for life. Some strategies for embracing sustainable habits include:

- Eating a balanced diet: Continue to prioritize nutrient-dense foods, including fruits, vegetables, lean proteins, and whole grains, while allowing for occasional treats in moderation.

- Staying active: Maintain a regular exercise routine that includes a variety of activities you enjoy, such as walking, cycling, strength training, or yoga.

- Practicing mindful eating: Stay attuned to hunger and fullness cues, savoring each bite and eating with intention rather than mindlessly.

- Managing stress: Incorporate stress management techniques such as meditation, deep breathing, or spending time in nature to support overall well-being.

- Getting enough sleep: Prioritize sleep hygiene and aim for seven to nine hours of quality sleep each night to support weight maintenance and overall health.

Building a Support System

Having a strong support system can make a significant difference in maintaining weight loss. Surround yourself with friends, family members, or a community of like-minded individuals who understand and support your goals. Share your successes, challenges, and strategies for staying on track, and lean on each other for encouragement and accountability.

Monitoring Progress and Adjusting as Needed

Regularly monitoring your progress and making adjustments as needed are essential for long-term weight maintenance. Keep track of your weight, measurements, and other markers of progress, such as energy levels, mood, and fitness performance. If you notice any changes or challenges, such as weight gain or increased cravings, assess your habits and make adjustments as necessary to get back on track.

Celebrating Milestones and Non-Scale Victories

While the number on the scale is one measure of progress, it's essential to celebrate other milestones and non-scale victories along the way. Whether it's fitting into a smaller clothing size, reaching a fitness milestone, or noticing improvements in energy levels or confidence, take time to acknowledge and celebrate your achievements.

Staying Flexible and Adaptable

Life is full of changes and challenges, and maintaining weight loss requires flexibility and adaptability. Be prepared to adjust your strategies and habits as needed in response to changes in your schedule, environment, or goals. Remember that consistency is key, but perfection is not required.

In summary, maintaining weight loss in the long term is a journey that requires commitment, patience, and flexibility. By setting realistic expectations, embracing sustainable habits, building a support system, monitoring progress, celebrating victories, and staying flexible and adaptable, you can achieve lasting success and enjoy the benefits of a healthy lifestyle for years to come. Remember that weight maintenance is not a destination but a lifelong journey, and with dedication and perseverance, you can navigate the ups and downs with confidence and resilience.

Chapter 10: Sustainable Habits for Long-Term Success

Achieving weight loss is a significant accomplishment, but maintaining those results in the long term requires adopting sustainable habits that support a healthy lifestyle. In this chapter, we'll explore the importance of sustainable habits, strategies for establishing them, and how they contribute to lasting success.

Understanding Sustainable Habits

Sustainable habits are behaviors and practices that can be maintained over the long term without feeling overly restrictive or burdensome. Unlike short-term fad diets or extreme exercise regimens, sustainable habits focus on making gradual, lasting changes that support overall health and well-being.

These habits prioritize balance, moderation, and enjoyment, allowing individuals to maintain their weight loss results without feeling deprived or overwhelmed.

Strategies for Establishing Sustainable Habits

Building sustainable habits requires a thoughtful and deliberate approach. Here are some strategies to help you establish habits that support long-term success:

- Set Realistic Goals: Start by setting realistic and achievable goals that align with your values and priorities. Break larger goals into smaller, more manageable steps, and celebrate your progress along the way.

- Focus on Behavior Change: Instead of solely focusing on outcomes such as weight loss or body measurements, concentrate on changing behaviors and habits that contribute to overall health. This could include eating more fruits and vegetables, being more active, or practicing portion control.

- Make Gradual Changes: Trying to revamp your whole lifestyle overnight is not tolerable. Instead, make small, incremental changes to your diet, exercise pattern, and lifestyle practices, allowing time for these changes to become ingrained and sustainable over time.

- Find Enjoyable Activities: Choose physical activities and exercises that you enjoy and look forward to, whether it's hiking, dancing, swimming, or playing a sport. If you enjoy what you're doing, you may probably cling to it in the long run.

- Practice Mindful Eating: Be aware of hunger and fullness cues, eat slowly, and taste each bite. Avoid distractions such as TV or smartphones during meals, and focus on enjoying the taste and texture of your food.

- Plan Ahead: Take time to plan your meals, snacks, and physical activities in advance. Having a plan in place can help you make healthier choices and avoid impulsive decisions.

- Build a Support System: Surround yourself with supportive friends, family members, or a community of like-minded individuals who understand and encourage your goals. Share your successes, challenges, and strategies for maintaining healthy habits.

- Be Flexible: Life is unpredictable, and there will be times when your routine is disrupted or you face unexpected challenges. Be flexible and adaptable, and don't let setbacks derail your progress. Instead, focus on finding alternative solutions and getting back on track as soon as possible.

The Benefits of Sustainable Habits

Establishing sustainable habits offers numerous benefits beyond weight loss, including:

- Improved Overall Health: Sustainable habits support overall health and well-being by promoting healthy eating, regular physical activity, and stress management.

- Increased Energy Levels: Adopting sustainable habits can boost energy levels, improve mood, and enhance cognitive function, allowing you to feel more vibrant and productive throughout the day.

- Enhanced Quality of Life: By prioritizing balance and moderation, sustainable habits allow you to enjoy a fulfilling and satisfying life without feeling restricted by rigid rules or limitations.

- Long-Term Weight Maintenance: Sustainable habits are key to maintaining weight loss results in the long term. By incorporating healthy behaviors into your daily routine, you can prevent weight regain and enjoy lasting success.

In summary, establishing sustainable habits is essential for long-term success on the weight loss journey. By focusing on gradual behavior change, making small, manageable adjustments to your lifestyle, and prioritizing balance, moderation, and enjoyment, you can create habits that support a healthy, fulfilling life for years to come. Remember that sustainable habits are not about perfection but about progress and consistency over time. By embracing sustainable habits and prioritizing your health and well-being, you can achieve lasting success and enjoy the many benefits of a healthier lifestyle.

Chapter 11: The Power of Self-Reflection and Continuous Improvement

Self-reflection is a powerful tool for personal growth and development, especially on the weight loss journey. In this chapter, we'll explore the importance of self-reflection, how it can enhance your weight loss efforts, and strategies for incorporating self-reflection into your routine for continuous improvement.

Understanding Self-Reflection

Self-reflection involves taking a step back to examine your thoughts, feelings, and behaviors with curiosity and honesty. It's an opportunity to gain insight into your motivations, strengths, and areas for growth, ultimately leading to greater self-awareness and empowerment.

Benefits of Self-Reflection in Weight Loss

Self-reflection can have numerous benefits for weight loss, including:

- Identifying patterns: Self-reflection allows you to recognize patterns in your eating, exercise, and lifestyle habits, helping you understand what's working well and what may need adjustment.
- Exploring triggers: By exploring your thoughts, emotions, and behaviors around food and exercise, you can identify triggers for overeating, emotional eating, or other challenges, allowing you to develop healthier coping strategies.
- Clarifying goals: Self-reflection helps you clarify your goals and motivations for weight loss, ensuring they are aligned with your values and priorities.
- Boosting motivation: Reflecting on your progress, accomplishments, and setbacks can boost motivation

and confidence, reminding you of how far you've come and inspiring you to keep moving forward.

- Fostering resilience: Self-reflection builds resilience by helping you develop a growth mindset, learn from setbacks, and bounce back stronger than before.

Strategies for Self-Reflection

Incorporating self-reflection into your routine doesn't have to be complicated. Below are some strategies to enable you get started:

- Journaling: Keep a journal to record your thoughts, feelings, and experiences related to your weight loss journey. Write about your successes, challenges, insights, and goals, and use your journal as a tool for self-discovery and growth.

- Mindful moments: Take time each day to pause and reflect on your experiences. This could be during a quiet moment in the morning, while out for a walk, or before bed. Practice mindfulness by adjusting your thinking, feelings, and bodily sensations without verdict.

- Regular check-ins: Schedule regular check-ins with yourself to assess your progress and identify areas for improvement. This could be weekly, monthly, or as needed, depending on your preferences and schedule.

- Feedback loop: Seek feedback from others, such as friends, family members, or a trusted mentor, to gain different perspectives on your progress and challenges. Open up to constructive criticism and benefit from it as an opportunity for development.

- Visualization: Use visualization techniques to imagine yourself achieving your goals and overcoming obstacles. Visualize the steps you need to take to reach your goals and the feelings of success and fulfillment that come with achieving them.

Embracing Continuous Improvement

The journey to weight loss is not linear, and there will inevitably be ups and downs along the way. Embrace the process of continuous improvement, focusing on progress rather than perfection. Each day puts forward a possibility to learn, grow, and become the best version of yourself.

In summary, self-reflection is a powerful tool for personal growth and development, especially on the weight loss journey. By taking the time to reflect on your thoughts, feelings, and behaviors, you can gain insight into your motivations, strengths, and areas for improvement. Incorporating self-reflection into your routine can enhance your weight loss efforts, boost motivation, and foster resilience for long-term success. Remember that self-reflection is a journey, not a destination, and with dedication and perseverance, you can continue to learn, grow, and thrive on your weight loss journey.

Appendix

Sample Meal Plans and Recipes

Here are some sample meal plans and recipes to help you get started on your weight loss journey:

Sample Meal Plan 1: Balanced and Nutritious

Breakfast:
- Scrambled eggs with spinach, tomatoes, and mushrooms
- Whole grain toast
- Fresh fruit salad (pineapple, berries, and melon)

Lunch:
- Grilled chicken salad with mixed greens, cherry tomatoes, cucumbers, and avocado
- Balsamic vinaigrette dressing

- Whole grain roll

Snack:

- Greek yogurt with honey and almonds

Dinner:

- Baked salmon with lemon and herbs
- Quinoa pilaf with roasted vegetables (bell peppers, zucchini, and onions)
- Steamed broccoli

Snack:

- Sliced apple with peanut butter

Sample Meal Plan 2: Plant-Based and Flavorful

Breakfast:

- Overnight oats with almond milk, chia seeds, sliced banana, and cinnamon
- Mixed nuts and seeds

Lunch:

- Chickpea and vegetable stir-fry with tofu
- Brown rice

Snack:

- Hummus with baby carrots and cucumber slices

Dinner:

- Lentil soup with kale and sweet potatoes
- Whole grain bread

Snack:

- Air-popped popcorn with nutritional yeast

Sample Meal Plan 3: Quick and Easy

Breakfast:

- Almond milk with whole grain cereal and sliced strawberries

- Hard-boiled egg

Lunch:

- Turkey and avocado wrap with lettuce, tomato, and mustard
- Baby carrots with hummus

Snack:

- Greek yogurt with granola

Dinner:

- Grilled shrimp skewers with bell peppers, onions, and cherry tomatoes
- Quinoa salad with cucumber, feta cheese, and lemon vinaigrette

Snack:

- Almond butter with rice cakes and slices of banana.

Sample Recipes:

Grilled Chicken Salad:

- Marinate chicken breast in olive oil, lemon juice, garlic, and herbs.

- Grill until cooked through and slice.

- Toss mixed greens with cherry tomatoes, cucumbers, avocado, and balsamic vinaigrette.

- Top salad with grilled chicken slices.

Lentil Soup:

- Sauté celery, carrots and onions in olive oil until it is soft.

- Add rinsed lentils, vegetable broth, diced tomatoes, kale, and sweet potatoes.

- Simmer until lentils and vegetables are tender.

- Season with salt, pepper, and herbs like thyme and rosemary.

Chickpea Stir-Fry:

- Sauté diced tofu in sesame oil until golden brown.
- Add sliced bell peppers, broccoli florets, and snap peas.
- Stir in cooked chickpeas and a sauce made from soy sauce, garlic, ginger, and a splash of rice vinegar.
- Serve over brown rice.

These sample meal plans and recipes provide a variety of options to suit different tastes and dietary preferences while supporting weight loss goals. Feel free to adjust portion sizes and ingredients to fit your individual needs and preferences. Remember to focus on whole, nutrient-dense foods and listen to your body's hunger and fullness cues. Enjoy your meals and happy cooking!

Exercise Routines for Beginners, Intermediate and Advanced Levels

Here are exercise routines tailored for beginners, intermediate, and advanced levels:

Beginner Exercise Routine:

Warm-Up:
- 5-10 minutes of light cardio (walking, jogging in place, or cycling)

Strength Training:
- Bodyweight squats: 2 sets of 10-12 reps
- Push-ups (modified or against a wall if needed): 2 sets of 8-10 reps
- Dumbbell rows (using light weights or household objects): 2 sets of 10-12 reps per arm
- Plank: Hold for 20-30 seconds

Cardiovascular Exercise:

- Brisk walking or jogging: 20-30 minutes

Cool Down:

- 5-10 minutes of stretching focusing on major muscle groups

Intermediate Exercise Routine:

Warm-Up:

- 5-10 minutes of light cardio (jumping jacks, high knees, or jump rope)

Strength Training:

- Goblet squats: 3 sets of 10-12 reps
- Push-ups: 3 sets of 8-10 reps
- Dumbbell chest press: 3 sets of 10-12 reps
- Perform bent-over rows for 3 sets, aiming for 10-12 repetitions each.

- Complete 3 sets of plank with leg lifts, doing 10 repetitions per leg.

Cardiovascular Exercise:
- Interval training (alternating between high-intensity bursts and recovery periods): 20-30 minutes (e.g., sprinting for 1 minute, walking for 2 minutes)

Cool Down:
- 5-10 minutes of stretching focusing on major muscle groups

Advanced Exercise Routine:

Warm-Up:
- 5-10 minutes of dynamic stretching or mobility exercises (arm circles, leg swings, etc.)

Strength Training:

- Barbell back squats: 4 sets of 6-8 reps

- Deadlifts: 4 sets of 6-8 reps

- Execute bench presses across 4 sets, aiming for 6-8 reps in each set.

- Pull-ups or lat pull-downs: 4 sets of 6-8 reps

- Romanian deadlifts: 3 sets of 8-10 reps

Cardiovascular Exercise:

- High-intensity interval training (HIIT) circuit: 20-30 minutes (e.g., alternating between sprints, burpees, jumping lunges, and kettlebell swings)

Cool Down:

- 10-15 minutes of static stretching targeting all major muscle groups, focusing on flexibility and mobility

Tips for Progression:

- Increase weight gradually as you get stronger and more comfortable with the exercises.

- Progressively increase the intensity and duration of cardiovascular exercises.

- Incorporate new exercises and variations to keep your workouts challenging and engaging.

- Pay attention to your body's signals and take breaks as necessary to avoid overtraining and injury.

- Stay consistent with your workouts and adjust your routine as needed based on your goals and progress.

Prior to beginning any new exercise regimen, particularly if you have existing health issues, seek advice from a healthcare provider. Additionally, consider working with a certified personal trainer to ensure proper form and technique, especially when performing more advanced exercises. Enjoy your workouts and stay committed to your fitness journey!

Glossary

1. Calorie: A unit of measurement for energy derived from food and beverages. Calories are either burned for energy or stored as fat in the body.

2. Macronutrients: Nutrients required in large amounts for proper growth, metabolism, and other bodily functions. The three main macronutrients are carbohydrates, proteins, and fats.

3. Micronutrients: Nutrients required in smaller amounts for various physiological processes, including vitamins and minerals.

4. Carbohydrates: Macronutrients found in foods like grains, fruits, vegetables, and dairy products. These are the major energy source for the body.

5. Proteins: Macronutrients essential for building and repairing tissues, synthesizing enzymes and hormones, and supporting immune function. Found in foods like meat, poultry, fish, beans, nuts, and dairy products.

6. Fats: Macronutrients that provide energy, support cell growth, protect organs, and help absorb certain vitamins. Sources of fatty foods are oils, butter, nuts, fatty fish, and avocados.

7. Fiber: A type of carbohydrate found in plant foods that aids in digestion, promotes satiety, and supports gut health.

8. Caloric Deficit: Consuming fewer calories than the body needs for maintenance, leading to weight loss.

9. Caloric Surplus: Consuming more calories than the body needs for maintenance, leading to weight gain.

10. Basal Metabolic Rate (BMR): The number of calories the body needs to maintain basic physiological functions while at rest.

11. Metabolism: The process by which the body converts food and beverages into energy. It includes basal metabolic rate (BMR), thermic effect of food (TEF), and physical activity.

12. Thermic Effect of Food (TEF): The energy expended by the body to digest, absorb, and metabolize nutrients from food.

13. Portion Control: Managing the amount of food consumed to maintain a healthy weight and prevent overeating.

14. Meal Prep: Planning and preparing meals in advance to save time, promote healthier eating habits, and support weight loss goals.

15. Plate Method: A visual guide for meal planning that involves dividing a plate into sections for different food groups, such as vegetables, proteins, and carbohydrates.

16. Glycemic Index (GI): A measure of how quickly carbohydrates in food raise blood sugar levels. Foods with a high GI cause a rapid spike in blood sugar, while those with a low GI cause a slower, more gradual increase.

17. Lean Body Mass (LBM): The weight of the body minus the weight of fat. It comprises of the muscles, organs, bones and water.

18. Body Mass Index (BMI): A measure of body fat based on height and weight. It is computed by weight in kilograms divided by height in meters squared.

19. Waist-to-Hip Ratio (WHR): A measure of body fat distribution calculated by dividing the waist circumference by the hip circumference. It is used to assess the risk of certain health conditions, including cardiovascular disease and diabetes.

20. Hydration: Maintaining adequate fluid balance in the body by consuming enough water and fluids throughout the day.

This glossary provides a basic understanding of commonly used terms in weight loss and nutrition. It's important to familiarize yourself with these terms to make informed decisions about your diet and lifestyle.